The Power of Images

How visualisation, art and dreams can change your life

Dr. Ruth Lever Kidson

Sphinx House

Published by Sphinx House Publishing, Norfolk
© Ruth Lever Kidson 2024

ISBN: 978-1-7393332-4-9

For Val Simanowitz
who was there at the start,
and for Frances Howlett
who encouraged me to write
this book

A NOTE ON TERMINOLOGY

In this book, I have used both 'patient' and 'client' to refer to people receiving therapy. This is because, while doctors, medical hypnotherapists, art therapists and psychoanalysts (such as Freud and Jung) use the term 'patient', humanistic therapists (as I discovered when I began my training) prefer the word 'client'.

Contents

When the power of the mind is mobilized for healing the body . . . it is as scientific as the appropriate use of antibiotics – *John E. Sarno (1923-2017) Professor of Rehabilitation Medicine, New York University School of Medicine*

The power of the mind is amazing, and we've barely scratched the surface of what it can do – *Charlie Sheen, actor*

Never underestimate the power of the mind – *Martin Pistorius, web designer who recovered from locked-in syndrome (pseudocoma) after12 years*

Power of mind is infinite – *Koichi Tohei (1920-2011) 10th Dan aikido master*

Chapter One

Introduction

The first time I came across the idea of the therapeutic use of images was in 1980. I was at a Health and Healing Conference run by the Wrekin Trust – an educational charity which had been set up nine years earlier. One of the speakers on this occasion was the American psychologist Stephanie Matthews-Simonton. She and her then husband, cancer specialist Dr. Carl Simonton, were making a name for themselves with a radical new approach to treating cancer in which they treated the mind and the body as a single entity, and in which visualisation played a large part.

I remember sitting spellbound as she told us about her work and talked about some of the patients she and her husband had treated. One, in particular, has always stayed in my mind. This was a man whose career had involved some fairly senior managerial roles. Now he had quite advanced bowel cancer and had signed up for the treatment program, which included 15 to 20 minutes of visualisation three times a day. He was told that, in these sessions, he was to picture the cancer cells, in whatever way he wanted to, and then picture his white blood cells (the body's defence system) working with his chemotherapy to destroy them.

This patient clearly had a romantic side to him because he decided to see his white blood cells as knights in white armour, riding on white chargers. The cancer cells he visualised were small, unpleasant animals that lived in a place that he called 'the cancer plain'. Each time he did his visualisation, he would picture himself blowing a horn to summon up countless battalions of white knights with white lances. And, with his managerial expertise, he gave each of them a quota to achieve each day. When he blew his horn a second time, they charged out onto the cancer plain and used their lances to spear enough cancer cells to meet their quota. Once they had done that, they rode to the far end of the cancer plain where the river of chemotherapy ran, and they dumped the cells they had caught into the stream where they dissolved and were swept away.

At first, the treatment seemed to be working well. But one day, the patient arrived in quite a distressed state. He had sounded his horn for the white knights to appear but, instead of coming in on huge white horses, they arrived riding white dogs – and the lack of height meant they were unable to use their lances to spear the cancer cells. The Simontons knew that, in the past, this patient had had occasional episodes of clinical depression and it seemed to them that, although he was not yet aware that he was slipping into another attack, his visualisation was sending him a warning. They prescribed some antidepressants and, before long, the knights returned on their sturdy white chargers.

On another occasion, when the knights responded to his summons they were carrying crooked lances so that, once again, it was impossible for them to spear the cancer cells. As part of the visualisation, the patient asked the knights why this had happened and was told that he needed to sort out some problems that were causing him stress at work. Once he had done this, all the knights returned with straight lances.

After this, all went well but, some months later, the patient came for his appointment in a very worried state. His knights were no longer bringing back their quota. However, on this occasion, it turned out that there was nothing for him to worry about. The reason there were so few cancer cells for the knights to kill was that the cancer had more or less disappeared. As time went on, he gradually reduced the knights' quota until the cancer had completely gone.

I remember, too, another case (although I can't recall whether Stephanie Simonton talked about it at the time or whether I read about it later on) in which a patient did so well with his visualisation, dissolving away his cancer, that he decided to try a similar technique with his arthritis and sent his white cells into his joints to smooth away the rough areas that were causing him pain. Against all expectations, it worked. The condition of his joints improved and he was able to walk easily again.

Three or four years after I went to the Health and Healing conference, I had the opportunity to train as a medical hypnotherapist. At the time, I was working as an Army medical officer which meant that the vast majority of my patients were fit young men. And it was my job to ensure that they stayed fit. But, at that time, about 50% of all young men smoked – and soldiers were no different. I knew that hypnotherapy could be used to help people to stop smoking, so I signed up for the course. What I didn't realise was that hypnotherapy could be an effective treatment for a wide range of medical and psychological conditions. And, as I discovered when I started my course, many of those treatments involved visualisation.

Around this time, too, people started to become aware of studies carried out in the Soviet Union which were showing how visualisation could improve the performance of athletes. Nowadays most top athletes practise some form of visualisation. Those who have been injured have found that recovery is speeded up and a return to their previous form occurs much more quickly if they picture themselves performing their sport and, in effect, reminding their muscles of what they have to do. I have read about athletes who have been bed-bound or in a cast for weeks on end and who, having worked with visualisation while they have been immobilised, have needed only a little physiotherapy to return them to peak condition once they are able to move around again.

Another technique used by athletes is known as emotive imagery, where they remember a positive emotional reaction to something. In an article in the Sport Journal (*Utilizing Imagery to Enhance Injury Rehabilitation*, Jan. 5th 2017), Marty Durden writes: "When an athlete associates a successful experience with one of the senses, it is easier to recall that event. For instance, an athlete has a great performance, and remembers that the pregame music contained a certain song. To stimulate another great performance, the athlete has only to replay this same song in his mind."

A number of years after I did my hypnotherapy training, I gave up clinical medicine and trained as a psychotherapist. Once again, it was the use of images and visualisation in therapy that particularly caught my attention. During the course of my career as a therapist I have used a range of visualisations – some of my own devising, others that I have adopted or adapted from techniques used by other people. And I never cease to be amazed at how effective they can be. An added bonus is that they don't just have to be confined to the therapy room – the patient can use the visualisation at home in order to help his or her treatment on its way.

In this book I have described the visualisations and other techniques that I use in the same way that I would explain them to a patient in the therapy room. I would suggest that you pick one that appeals to you and that seems appropriate for you and use it every day for a week or two before trying anything else. As you become more comfortable with a visualisation, it should become easier and more effective. But if you're not comfortable with it, give it up and try a different one. Not every visualisation suits everyone. I remember being on a course a number of years ago when the tutor took us on a guided visualisation in which we went up in a hot air balloon. The visualisation was meant to be restful – but I don't like heights and I found it profoundly uncomfortable.

Once you have found one or two visualisations that you like, continue with them until they have done the job you set them. And then continue with them once or twice a week, just as maintenance.

The second section of this book deals with physical images – either ones that we choose to look at or ones that we draw ourselves. These can be used to express our emotions but can also help us to untangle our thoughts and our feelings in order to make them easier to deal with.

The third section deals with dreams. Sometimes our dreams are a simple reflection of what is going on in our lives at present but, at other times, they may be giving us clues about what we need to know or to do in order to progress.

One final word of caution. Self help is a wonderful thing, but if you have emotional problems that are overwhelming, please seek help. There are a number of counselling and psychotherapy websites that list only fully qualified therapists and which give details of each therapist so that you can decide which one might suit you. You will find a list of websites at the end of this book. Asking help from a therapist does not in any way imply failure on your part – after all, if your bath sprung a leak you'd call a plumber (unless you, yourself, are a plumber) and if you lost tiles off your roof you'd call in a roofer (unless that's your particular area of expertise). A therapist has done years of training and is there not only to offer you a safe space in which you can talk about your problems but to help you to find your way out of them.

PART ONE

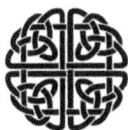

VISUALISATION

Chapter Two

What if I Can't Visualise?

A lot of people think they can't visualise – I used to be one of them. But if you have ever daydreamed – which most of us have – or if you have ever had a dream – which all of us have – it means that your brain is capable of producing images that aren't just to do with what your eyes are telling it.

If you have difficulty visualising, don't worry about it. You can still do the exercises in this section of the book. But instead of trying to visualise something, just allow yourself to imagine it. So, for example, if the exercise asks you to picture yourself walking along a path in the countryside on a glorious summer's day, you may find that you can't see it in your mind. But perhaps you can remember a walk in the country that you took at some time in the past, and you may be able to remember how it felt – the warmth of the sun on your skin, the light breeze cooling the air, the long grass brushing against your ankles. Or perhaps you remember the smells – the scent of the grass and of the wild flowers, or other 'country smells' indicating that there are farm animals nearby. Or maybe it is your sense of hearing that is strongest and you can recall hearing the slight swishing sound of the breeze in the trees, the song of the birds flying overhead or the mooing of cows in the distance. And, if you can't remember a walk in the country, you could just try imagining what it would *be* like without worrying about what it would *look* like. All our senses can tell us things so, if you can't visualise at first, just use the other senses and, you never know, the ability to visualise may just creep up on you!

However, there is an exercise that may help you. It is what took me from being unable to visualise to being able to visualise things in brilliant colour in one fell swoop. At the time I was in a personal development group run by Gestalt psychologist Mary Hykel-Hunt. On this particular day she told us that we were going to use tattwas to enhance our ability to visualise. I can't remember how she explained tattwas to us, but Wikipedia describes them as "the elements or aspects of reality that constitute human experience . . . according to various Indian schools of philosophy". The number of tattwas varies according to which school of philosophy you follow but Mary introduced us to the Hindu tantric system which has just five. Each has its own symbol:

- A yellow square that represents Earth

- A blue circle that represents Air

- A red triangle that represents Fire

- A silver crescent that represents Water

- And a black oval that represents Spirit

She asked us to pick one and then to close our eyes, relax and imagine that the symbol we had picked had become a doorway through which we could step. And, once through the door, we were free to wander around whatever we found on the other side. Knowing my problems with visualisation, Mary then suggested that, rather than try to visualise the shape of the symbol-doorway that I had chosen, I should try to feel it. So, having shut my eyes, I imagined that I was using my hands to feel around the shape of the silver crescent. I remember that it felt like wood and was rough in places. I felt carefully around the whole crescent shape – and then I stepped through it.

What happened next was amazing. I found myself in field of corn. I could see it clearly, and I could see a farmhouse a little way away. I walked along a path that led to the house and let myself in through a door which led straight into a large kitchen with a big wooden table in the centre. There were chairs around the table and, on one of them, a large ginger cat was sleeping.

Having looked around the kitchen, I went out through another door which opened onto another path. Following the path, I walked slowly up a steep hill, finally reaching a small flat area. Looking over to my left I could see a scene stretching out before me which reminded me of those atmospheric Oriental drawings that depict mountains half covered in mists. I stretched out my hands towards the view – and rainbows came pouring out of my finger tips. At which point, Mary told us it was time to come back into the room.

Since this extraordinary experience, I have always been able to visualise. Sometimes the details are clear, at other times less so. But I can always picture something. So, if you have difficulty visualising, I would recommend trying this exercise. These are the steps:

- Pick one of the tattwa shapes - a yellow square, a blue circle, a red triangle, a silver crescent or a black oval

- Close your eyes and relax.

- Imagine that you are standing next to a doorway which is one of the tattwa shapes and that you are running your hands around its the inner rim. Can you feel what it is made of? Is it smooth and cool, suggesting metal? Is it slightly rough, indicating wood? Does it feel like plastic? Or is it made from a more unusual material – maybe it is formed from jelly, or it could be a living plant, or perhaps the shape is covered in fur. Just relax and go where your imagination takes you.

- Once you have a clear idea of what the doorway feels like, step through – and just see what happens.

If you do the exercise and are able to get an impression of what the doorway feels like, but nothing happens when you step through, leave it for a little while and then try it again with a different shape. While it is impossible to guarantee that individual exercises will work for everyone, sometimes just adjusting a few of the details will bring the results you want.

Chapter Three

Let's Start by Relaxing

You will notice that, when describing visualisation techniques, I mention right at the start the need to relax. However, this is something that a lot of us find difficult. So here are a couple of visualisations that I use with my clients to help them to relax. The golden light visualisation aids physical relaxation, while the swim at sunrise is useful if you need to calm your mind. You might like to have someone read the instructions to you, or perhaps record yourself reading the instructions – but, in either case, make sure that you leave plenty of time between the steps. Ideally, allow about ten to fifteen minutes for either exercise.

THE GOLDEN LIGHT

- Make yourself comfortable, then shut your eyes.

- Now lift one of your hands and touch the crown of your head with your finger. Press firmly so that, after you take your finger away, you can still feel the spot that you pressed.

- Rest your hand back on your lap.

- Now focus on that spot on top of your head and imagine that a warm, golden light is pouring down onto it. See if you can feel the warmth.

- Then allow the light to spread over your scalp, gently soothing away any tensions.

- When you are ready, let the light flow down onto your forehead. Again, let it soothe away any tightness. Feel the muscles in your forehead starting to relax.

- Next, be aware of the light flowing down over the rest of your face, working its magic on all the muscles. Feel it gently soothing your eyelids so that your eyes feel relaxed. Be aware of it moving over your jaw, taking away any tightness and allowing your jaw to become slack.

- And now let this lovely warm, honey-coloured light flow down into your neck. The neck is an area that frequently becomes tense so just feel the light gently massaging away any tensions, allowing your head to feel comfortably balanced.

- Then, when you are ready, let the light flow into your shoulders. Take your time here – most of us have tense shoulders. Just allow the light to do its work, gently soothing away tensions so that the muscles in your shoulders start to relax and go loose.

- And now allow the light to flow down your arms and into your hands, right to the tips of your fingers. As it does its work, gently soothing away all the tensions, you may become aware that your arms are starting to feel quite heavy with relaxation.

- Next, this beautiful, warm honey-coloured light is going to spread even further, softly circling your chest so that your breathing becomes very gentle, almost as though you were asleep. And let the light flow down your back and into your hips. Feel yourself sinking into your chair, as though you were sitting on the softest of cushions.

• Then allow the light to flood across your abdomen, helping you to let go of any tensions there, soothing any muscle tightness and allowing you to relax even more. You may be aware of your intestines gurgling as a result of your new ability to relax.

• And finally, let the light flow down your legs and into your feet, right to the tips of your toes. The muscles in your thighs have to work so hard when you stand and when you walk or run. Just allow the light to massage them gently so that they soften and relax. And then do the same with your calves, which also have to work hard whenever you stand or move your legs. Feel all that tightness dissolving and your legs starting to feel heavy with relaxation.

• Now take a few minutes just to enjoy this lovely feeling of relaxation as the warm, golden light flows around your entire body. And then, when you are ready, in your own time, very, very gently open your eyes and come back into the room.

A SWIM AT SUNRISE

- Make yourself comfortable, then shut your eyes.

- Now imagine that you are standing on a beautiful sandy beach at sunrise. There is no one else in sight. The sand is soft beneath your feet and, as you look around, you can see the trees that surround the little cove where you are standing. You can hear the dawn chorus of birds as they greet the sun which is starting to rise up out of the sea.

- The sea itself is very calm and clear and you walk down the beach into the water which feels warm on your feet.

- When you are ready, walk further into the water and start to swim towards the sunrise. You swim effortlessly, enjoying the feel of the water on your skin. As you swim, you are aware of the sun slowly rising over the horizon.

- As the sun rises, you begin to feel its warmth, and its rays start to relax and to invigorate you. You are aware that you are swimming strongly, with confidence and with enjoyment.

- Continue to swim and to enjoy the water and the peace you are starting to feel. When you are ready, turn around and swim back to the beach. Notice how the sun is starting to light up the sand and the trees and how it is sparkling off the water.

- As you walk out of the sea, the sun dries the water from your skin, making it feel clean and fresh. On the beach you see a lounger chair, with soft, comfortable cushions. When you reach it, lie down on it and then slowly let the scene fade from your mind before you gently open your eyes and come back into the room.

Chapter Four

Visualisations for Apprehension and Difficult Situations

Have you ever felt apprehensive about something you had to do – give a speech, take an exam, or go for an interview, for example? Or perhaps you have had colleagues who you didn't get on with, and having to work with them was stressful. These are both things that many people encounter at one time or another.

Here are two visualisations that I frequently recommend to my clients in order to overcome these feelings. The first is more specific to a particular situation than the second, as you will see.

METHOD ONE

- Start, as usual, by making yourself comfortable, shutting your eyes and relaxing. Now allow yourself to think back to a situation where you felt confident and fully in control of what was going on. If it is something that you do every day, such as driving a car, think back to how you felt when you first mastered a particular manoeuvre, or when you passed your test. Or perhaps there was a particular event when you achieved something that gave you pleasure – maybe you won a competition or baked a delicious cake or finished a difficult piece of work.

- Now concentrate on that event and allow your feeling of satisfaction to grow. Know that you did well and acknowledge that in a similar situation you would certainly do well again. Feel that confidence in your own abilities in that particular situation, and let the feeling grow.

- Once you can feel that strong confidence within yourself, ask your subconscious mind to give you an image to represent that feeling. Don't think about it or try to force it. Just put out the thought to your subconscious mind and then continue to concentrate on the feeling of confidence.

- The image that your subconscious mind gives you could be anything – from a peaceful landscape to a cup and saucer to a pink elephant! Take a note of it, then gently open your eyes and come back into the room.

Now when you go into a situation that requires some confidence or courage, all you have to do is to remember the image which will then act as a trigger to bring back that strong feeling of confidence. When I tried this visualisation, I got an image of a brightly coloured beach ball. So when, a few days later, I had to deal with a situation that was making me nervous, I went in to it with an imaginary beach ball tucked under my arm – and it worked!

METHOD TWO

This was taught to me, years ago, by another therapist, Judith O'Hagan. I have used it myself to good effect and a lot of my clients, to whom I have taught it, have found it helpful as well.

- Start, as always, by making yourself comfortable, shutting your eyes and relaxing.

- Now imagine that you are wearing a cloak. It is made from a beautiful soft, dark blue velvet and is very comfortable to wear. It is really long, just touching the floor when you stand up. And it fits snuggly around your neck. It is very roomy and the fabric overlaps in front, so all your body is covered.

- The cloak has a hood, too, which covers all of your head apart from your face. And both the cloak and the hood are lined with a lovely, light, silky fabric.

- Inside the cloak is *your* space. Nothing can get through the cloak except love – going in or going out. If anything should happen while you are wearing your cloak that might in normal circumstances upset you or make you feel anxious, the cloak will protect you and keep you feeling loved and protected.

I suggest that you practise visualising the cloak for five

to ten minutes every day until you get to the point where all that you have to do is to think of the cloak and it will be there. Then, if something happens and you need it, you can just call it up and you will be protected within seconds.

Chapter Five

Another
Visualisation to
Treat Anxiety

This is a method that I learned when I was training as a medical hypnotherapist and while, ideally, it should be used with the patient in a hypnotic trance, it can also be used by someone in a state of relaxation. A lot of mystical mumbo jumbo has been talked about hypnosis in the past but, in fact, it is simply a state of extreme relaxation. There are, too, degrees of hypnosis – it is not necessary for a patient to be in a really deep state for the treatment to work. Some techniques can work just as well when the patient is in a very light hypnotic trance.

With this in mind, I started to use some hypnosis techniques with psychotherapy clients who were not hypnotised but who had learned to relax. And I discovered that, although they might take a little longer to work, the techniques could still be effective. This is one of them.

This technique is best used when the cause of the anxiety is something very specific – for example, if you suffer from a fear of flying or a fear of spiders. I have used it successfully with clients who suffered, among other things, from claustrophobia and from dental phobia.

Before you try it, I suggest that you familiarise yourself with the golden light relaxation technique described in chapter three and the cloak technique described in chapter four, as these can both be used in conjunction with the present exercise and, if you have practised them, they should help to make this exercise more effective.

Because this technique is specific to the user's fear, I am going to give the instructions that I would give to someone suffering from agoraphobia (fear of open spaces) who starts to become anxious as soon as he opens his front door.

- As usual, make yourself comfortable, shut your eyes and relax. Use the golden light relaxation exercise to ensure that you are fully relaxed before going any further.

- Once you are nicely relaxed imagine that you are in a film that can be paused or can be run forwards or backwards as desired. And imagine that you are at home and standing by the front door. Check on how you are feeling. Are you still relaxed? If so, open the front door a fraction. If not, use the cloak visualisation, allowing the cloak to protect you as you move forward in the exercise. If necessary, imagine the golden light filling the interior of the cloak, helping you to relax more. Then, once you are feeling comfortable, try opening the door again.

- When you have the door open a crack, check again on how you are feeling. If you are reasonably comfortable, open the door a fraction more. Continue to open it until you are aware of the anxiety returning. Then immediately pause the film and rewind it to a point where you feel comfortable again. If you haven't yet put on your cloak, do so, and reinforce your relaxation by directing the golden light to any parts of your body that feel tense.

- Allow yourself time to relax and then, when you are ready, try opening the door a little more. As soon as you feel the slightest bit of anxiety, pause the film. But this time, don't rewind it just yet. You know that you can so, hopefully, that will make you feel safe. But, for the moment, just see if you can tolerate this slight degree of anxiety. As soon as you feel it is too much, rewind the film as before.

- But if you find that you can tolerate this mild anxiety, see if you can reduce it by allowing the golden light to relax your body. And then see what happens if you open the door a little bit more.

- Continue in this way, pausing as soon as you feel anxious, relaxing and, if you are able to get the door fully open, seeing if you can take a step or two outside, until you feel you have gone as far as you can. It is very important that you don't push yourself too far. Always pause as soon as you feel anxious and only move forward again if you have been able to relax. If it gets uncomfortable at any time, rewind immediately to a place where you feel safe. And always rewind to that place at the end of the exercise, before opening your eyes.

As I said above, this technique can be used for dental phobia (visualising the journey to the dentist, going into reception and, in time, going in to see the dentist and having treatment), and for claustrophobia (stepping onto a bus or a train or an aeroplane or whatever causes your claustrophobia, with the doors still open, then gradually moving further down the carriage and allowing the doors to close). Always remember to pause and rewind if you feel uncomfortable.

You can adapt the technique to work with any number of fears. For example, if you have a fear of spiders, you could visualise a small spider on the wall on the opposite side of a large room, with someone standing ready to capture it in a glass, and then slowly, over time, increase the size of the spider – and, eventually, see yourself wielding the glass and catching it.

Obviously, in order to work, this is an exercise that needs to be repeated regularly, preferably every day. In time you will find that you will be able to do more and more in your imagination. Be aware, however, that doing something in your imagination doesn't necessarily mean that you will be able to do it as well in reality – at first. But constant practice should eventually bring you to the point where you can do in real life what you you have been visualising in the exercise.

Chapter Six

Cleansing and Clearing

There are times in all our lives that we feel we are being swamped – by work, by emotions, by demands on our time and by expectations that are being put on us by others. And sometimes it's very hard just to let things go. There are, however, three visualisations that can be very helpful in such situations.

THE WATERFALL

This is a gentle visualisation that can help you to relax at the end of an exhausting day, or a day on which you've been surrounded by other people who have encroached on your space.

- Close your eyes and relax. Then imagine that you are standing in front of a beautiful waterfall, with trees in full leaf to either side of you. The sky is clear blue and the waterfall shimmers in the sunshine. Around you, you can hear birds singing.

- Step into the waterfall. It feels very gentle on your skin but cool and refreshing.

- Allow the water to pour down, washing away all your tensions and anxieties.

- As you stand there, the waterfall may change colour. When it does so, it may feel a little different. Don't try to change the colour yourself – just notice and enjoy the colours you are being given.

- Once you feel completely cleansed and refreshed, step out of the waterfall and feel the sun drying your skin.

- When you are ready, very gently, open your eyes and come back into the room.

CUTTING CORDS

This visualisation is for those situations when you want to move forward and someone else is trying to hold you back. Perhaps you have broken up with your boyfriend or girlfriend and he or she wants to get back together although you know in your heart it would be a mistake. Or perhaps you want to apply for another job and your boss is trying to persuade you to stay. In those situations where a lot of pressure is being put on you, it can sometimes be hard to resist and you can end up going against your better judgement. This visualisation can reinforce your determination to do what you know is right for you.

- Close your eyes and relax. Then focus on your solar plexus. This is the area of your upper abdomen just under the V of your ribs. Often if we get a sudden shock, we will feel a tightening in the solar plexus. It is also the place that can feel uncomfortable when we are very nervous.

- Imagine that, running out of your solar plexus, are several cords – it doesn't matter how many – and these are attaching you to the person who is putting pressure on you.

- Be aware of how the cords seem to be pulling you towards that person.

- In your mind, explain kindly to that person why it is important that he or she should let you go.

- Then imagine that you are taking a large pair of golden scissors and, very carefully and with great compassion, cut through the cords. It is very important to do this with compassion, because the person on the other end of the cords is not trying to hurt you but is distressed at having to let you go.

- Once you have cut the cords, thank the person for allowing you to set yourself free.

- Then, in your own time, very gently open your eyes and come back into the room.

At first, if there are a lot of cords, you may not be able to cut them all in one go, so just cut as many as you can. And, as cords can grow back, you will probably have to do this visualisation a number of times before you feel completely free of the pressure that is being put on you. So I suggest that you repeat it daily until the situation is resolved.

THE GOLDEN CORD

This visualisation is one that I have adapted from a technique I read about many years ago in *The Psychic Healing Book* by Amy Wallace and Bill Henkin (now out of print). It is valuable for those times when you feel that things or people are crowding in on you or when you feel overwhelmed by what is going on in your life.

There used to be an advertisement on television – for a dry cleaning company, I think – where we were shown someone wearing a smart dark-coloured outfit which then turned white, so that we could see all the stains and the dirt that had attached itself to the fabric. This visualisation is similar in that we imagine all the stresses and strains of our daily life as a sort of sludge that has attached itself to us and needs to be washed away.

- Make yourself comfortable, close your eyes and relax. Then focus on a point in your body just in front of the base of your spine. And imagine that, curled up tightly in that place, is a golden cord. It is rather like one of those tape measures that come in cases – you pull out the tape when you want to measure something and then you press a button and the tape slides back into its case.

- Focus on the curled up golden cord, then run it out, as you would a tape measure, and allow it to run down from your body into whatever you are sitting or lying on, then through that down to the floor, through the floor and right down through the building, into the foundations. From there it continues to run down into the earth and then on and on until it reaches the centre of the earth, where it anchors itself.

- Now imagine that you have an extra pair of hands. They are not attached to your body (although they are controlled by you) so they can go wherever you send them. Imagine them going all round your body, scooping up all the sludge that the stresses and strains of life have left there. And, as they scoop it up, they are going to push it, gently, into the golden cord which will act as a waste-disposal. So all the sludge will flow swiftly down to where the cord is anchored at the centre of the earth and it will disperse and be neutralised so that it can't cause any harm.

- Continue doing this until your extra pair of hands has scooped up as much as it can and pushed it down the cord. Then draw up through the cord some clean, fresh, bubbling energy. Allow the energy to wash through you and around you, absorbing the bits of sludge that your hands couldn't reach. Then allow it to flow back down the cord to the centre of the earth where it will disperse and be neutralised.

- Repeat this step – bringing up clean, fresh, bubbling energy, using it to wash through you and around you, and then flushing it down the cord to be neutralised – as many times as you want to.

- Then, when you are ready, bring up one final lot of bubbling energy which you will keep for yourself.

- When you have done this, release the anchor which is holding the cord at the centre of the earth and allow the cord to retract through the earth, through the building in which you are, through whatever you are sitting or lying on, back into your body where it curls up in its original position in front of the base of your spine, so it will be available whenever you want to use it again.

- Then, when you are ready, gently open your eyes and slowly come back into the room.

Chapter Seven

A Little Bit of Mindfulness

Nowadays we hear a lot about mindfulness and how we should try to cultivate it. But many clients I talk to aren't quite sure how to begin. And so – because mindfulness can be so valuable – I am including this exercise here although, strictly speaking, it is not a visualisation.

I have had quite a number of clients over the years who are troubled by intrusive thoughts – thoughts that go round and round in their heads and that take them deeper and deeper down into depression and despair. Practising mindfulness can nip this vicious circle in the bud – and I know at least one person who was able to treat her recurrent depression using this alone. This is not to say, of course, that other forms of treatment should be rejected if recommended by a health professional. Always be guided by your doctor or your therapist. But mindfulness may help to speed up recovery from depression when it is accompanied by intrusive thoughts and may help to prevent recurrence.

AN EXERCISE FOR DEVELOPING MINDFULNESS

Unlike the other exercises in this book, you don't start by relaxing – although it is important that you are comfortable.

- Sit in an upright chair and try to ensure that your back is straight and that your body feels balanced. You may find it helpful to move your legs so that your knees are facing outwards, with the seat of your chair and your feet, seen from above, forming an equal sided triangle.

- Now shut your eyes and focus on your breathing. Don't alter it in any way – just observe it. Be aware of how your chest or your abdomen rise and fall with each breath. See if you can feel the air entering and leaving your nostrils. Try not to be distracted by anything else. Just focus on your breathing.

- Then, after half a minute or so, turn your attention to your scalp. How does it feel? Are you aware of any sensations – itching, tensions, discomfort? If so, don't try to do anything about them, but just observe them. Then, what about your ears? Can you feel anything there? Do they feel warm or cold? Is your hair brushing across them, and, if so, can you feel it? Are there any other sensations?

- And then return your attention to your breathing for half a minute or so.

- Now turn your attention to your face. How does it feel? Are you aware of any tensions or other sensations? Again, just observe. How do your eyes feel? Are they relaxed? And what about your eyelids? Then turn your attention to your jaw. Does it feel loose or tight? Are your teeth clamped together? And your mouth – are your lips closed or apart? Whereabouts in your mouth is your tongue? Is it touching your lower teeth or your upper teeth, or is it curled back in your mouth? Does your mouth feel moist or dry? Do you feel the need to swallow? Is there any discomfort in your mouth? Take your time to explore what you are feeling and experiencing.

- And then return your attention to your breathing for half a minute or so.

- Now turn your attention to your neck, shoulders and arms. As before, allow yourself to become aware of any sensations you can feel. Can you feel your clothes touching your skin? Where can you feel it most clearly? Is your neck straight or is your head drooping? Don't try to change anything – just observe. Are your arms relaxed or are you holding them stiffly? And where are your hands? Are the palms facing down or up? Are your fingers curved or straight? If you're wearing a watch or a bracelet or a ring, can you feel it on your skin? Take your time to explore what you are feeling and experiencing.

- And then return your attention to your breathing for half a minute or so.

- Next, turn your attention to your back. Are you sitting upright or are you slouching? Is your back comfortable or are there tensions? Are you leaning against the chair back – and, if so, can you feel the pressure of it on your skin? What about the seat of the chair? Are you aware of how it is supporting you? Is it comfortable or does it feel hard? And where, exactly, are you feeling the pressure?

- And then return your attention to your breathing for half a minute or so.

- Now start to focus on your abdomen. Are the muscles tense or relaxed? Are you wearing a belt or a piece of clothing with a waistband? Can you feel it? Are you aware of any sensations or discomfort within your abdomen. Whereabouts are they? As before, take your time to explore what you are feeling and experiencing.

- And then return your attention to your breathing for half a minute or so.

- Finally, turn your attention to your legs. Are they relaxed or are you aware of certain muscles feeling tense? Can you feel your clothes touching your skin? Are your feet flat on the ground? Are they comfortable. Can you feel your shoes pressing on your feet? Take your time exploring this last section of your body.

- And then, for one last time, return your attention to your breathing.

- After half a minute or so (it can be more, if you like) very gently and slowly open your eyes and come back into the room.

If you continue to practise until you find it relatively easy to keep focused on each part of the exercise in turn, you may like to try another exercise which is simpler – but also more difficult! It comes from the Buddhist tradition and is known as mindfulness of breathing.

In this exercise, you sit, as before, with your back straight and your body balanced. But, unlike the previous exercise, you keep your focus on your breathing throughout. And you count your breaths. So (in your head, not aloud) you say 'one' as you exhale the first breath, then 'two' as you exhale the second, and so on. It is very important that you don't try to change your breathing in any way but, rather that you just act as an observer. When you get to ten, you start again at one.

However . . . you will find that it is quite hard to get to ten without your mind wandering off.   When a thought comes into your mind, acknowledge it as a thought and let it go – and then start counting again from one. Many people find that they have to practise for quite a while before they can get to ten.

Like any exercise, the more you practise mindfulness, the easier it will become – I would suggest that you try to find time to do it every day if you can. If you do, you will, in time start to become more aware both of the world around you and also of your own thought processes. It is an exercise that is worth practising because not only does it allow you more control over your thoughts and feelings but, as one person said to me, "it makes all the colours of the world seem brighter".

USING MINDFULNESS TO OVERCOME INTRUSIVE THOUGHTS

One of the problems with intrusive thoughts is that they can take over, not allowing you the chance to challenge them before they drag you down to a point where you can't think of anything else, and they can make you thoroughly miserable. However, if you have been practising mindfulness, you can nip this vicious circle in the bud – as a number of my clients have found.

Once you are reasonably adept at mindfulness your mind will find it much harder to catch you unawares. This is particularly so if you have been practising mindfulness of breathing and have grown used to acknowledging thoughts as they come into your mind, and then dismissing them. Then, at any time – not just when you are practising – if an intrusive thought comes into your mind, you will be immediately aware of it and of the need to deal with it.

First of all, recognise it for what it is. Is it a criticism of yourself? Intrusive thoughts often are. If it is, ask yourself if it is a valid criticism (intrusive thoughts often aren't) or are you beating yourself up about something? If someone else had done what you are criticising yourself for, would you criticise them as harshly? If the answer to this is no, allow yourself to let go of the thought, just as you let go of thoughts when you are practising mindfulness.

If, however, you feel that the criticism is justified, ask yourself "Is there something I can do about it?" If the answer is no, acknowledge this and ask yourself "What have I learned from this that will be of value in the future?". And when you have an answer to that, acknowledge that we all make mistakes and that this is the way we learn. Then let go of the thoughts, knowing that you have moved on.

On the other hand, if the answer to your question as to whether there is something you can do about it is yes, ask yourself "Can I do it now?" and, if the answer is no, decide on what you can do and when. Then let the thoughts go until it is time to act on your decision.

If, rather than a criticism, the intrusive thought is a worry or anxiety, ask yourself "Is it relevant to what I'm doing now?" and, if the answer is no, let it go. If it is relevant, ask yourself what you can do about it and, if necessary, who you can ask to help you.

The point of working in this way is to train your mind not to descend into a state where thoughts are going round and round without any results other than making you feel bad. If you can identify the thought for what it is, as soon as it comes into your mind, you will be much better placed to be able to deal with it in a practical way.

Chapter Eight

What's Stopping Me?

M any of us have experienced a situation where, despite wanting to do something, we feel that there is something stopping us. We tell ourselves that we are not capable of doing it, we find excuses why we can't do it today or next week or next month, or we conveniently 'forget about it'. But what is it that is really holding us back? It is not that we don't want to do it – we can see all the advantages of taking this course of action and perhaps we have even dreamed about what life will be like afterwards. But we still sit on our hands and don't do anything about it.

And then there are other situations where we work really hard at something we are sure we can do, but somehow we just can't seem to get it right. Are we right in believing we can do it, or should we just admit defeat and turn our energies to other things?

There is a visualisation that can be very effective in telling us exactly what it is that is making us hesitate or that is stopping us from achieving what we believe we are capable of. And once we are consciously aware of that, it is often not too difficult to deal with it so that we can start to move forwards.

- Make yourself comfortable, close your eyes and relax. If necessary, use the golden light visualisation to ensure that you are truly relaxed.

- Imagine that you are walking along a little path in the middle of the countryside on a beautiful summer's day. There is no one else about and it all feels very peaceful.

- Be aware of what is around you – can you feel the warmth of the sun? And perhaps there is a soft breeze, ensuring that you don't get too hot. Are there birds singing? Is their song coming from a particular direction, or are they, perhaps, flying overhead?

- What is the countryside like? Is it very green or

does it seem a bit brown thanks to a hot spell? Are there flowers growing in the grass? What colours are they? Are there any trees? Are they close by or in the distance? Can you see any animals?

- As you walk, you will notice that, ahead of you, there is a little hill. The path that you are on goes up the hill a little way and then curves round it, so that you can't see where it leads to. Continue along the path and follow it up the hill.

- As you start to go up the hill, you know that something important waits for you around the bend. When you get there you will see, lying on the path in front of you, something that will give you a clue as to what is stopping you from moving forward with the project that you have been putting off or that has stalled.

- Don't think about what this object might be – just accept that it will be there, once you have reached the other side of the hill. And keep walking until it comes into view.

- Once you see the object, take time to look at it and understand what it is. Its significance may not be obvious immediately (although it often is). Take note of any details and commit the object to memory. Rarely, the object may make you feel uncomfortable or anxious (this happened to me, as I relate below). If this happens, remind yourself that you are perfectly safe and then look around you and you will see something else that will be there to help you and protect you.

- When you have finished inspecting the object, thank it for showing itself to you and very gently and slowly, open your eyes and come back into the room.

I clearly remember the first time I used this visualisation myself. I had recently started training for something that I was very keen to do. But I was lagging behind all the other people on the course. No matter how helpful the tutor and no matter how hard I tried, I couldn't do what I was being asked to do and yet there didn't seem to be any obvious reason why I was failing. So when Mary Hykel-Hunt, a Gestalt psychologist and the leader of the personal development group I went to at that time, suggested to the group that we try this visualisation to resolve any blocks we currently had, it seemed like the perfect opportunity to explore what was going wrong.

I visualised the path and the lovely countryside I was walking through, listening to the birds singing as I went along. The sun was warm and the breeze was pleasant. I followed the path up the hill and round the bend, expecting to see something lying there that would give me a clue. But there wasn't anything. There wasn't even a path. It ended in a steep drop down to the valley a long way below.

Now I don't like heights – I really don't like them. And I must have let out a little yelp as I visualised myself backing away from the edge. I remember Mary saying "It's OK, you're perfectly safe". And, when my facial expression obviously conveyed to her that I didn't feel very safe, she said "Look down at the ground and you'll see something that will help you to cope". I looked down - and there on the ground was a large pile of mountaineering equipment. And that made me laugh. Because the message was clear. What was holding me back from succeeding on my course was fear – fear that I couldn't do it. But I actually had all the equipment I needed – symbolised by the pile of crampons, ice picks, helmet and ropes – to make sure that I did succeed. Once I realised this I opened my eyes and came back.

From that point on, I found the course easier and I

had soon caught up with some of the others. At this point, I did the visualisation again, just to see if things had changed. They had. Instead of the sheer drop of the first visualisation, the path now continued down into the valley. It was very steep but it would be possible to negotiate it with good hiking boots and walking sticks. At the end of the course, when I had become as proficient as the others who were training with me, I did the visualisation yet again. This time, not only was there no sheer drop, but the path was no longer steep and I was able to stroll down the gentle slope into the valley.

Chapter Nine

Making Choices

It is not always easy to make choices. Sometimes the options facing us seem to have equally valid positive and negative aspects. We may spend sleepless nights and anxious days worrying about what to do and, when we finally decide on one of the options, we may be left with some doubt as to whether, in fact, we should have chosen the other one.

This visualisation helps us to make a more informed choice because it puts us in touch with how we feel subconsciously about the options and can reveal to us just why one feels better than the other. The technique was taught to me by Gestalt psychologist Mary Hykel-Hunt when I was in her personal development group, although I have changed it slightly over the years.

- Make yourself comfortable, shut your eyes and relax.

- Now, rest your hands on your thighs and turn them palm upwards. Make sure they are not touching each other.

- In your right hand imagine a puddle of colour that represents one of your options. Don't think about what colour it will be, but just allow it to appear and to become clear in your mind.

- Do the same with your left hand – allow a puddle of a different colour to appear, representing your second option. Let it become clear in your mind.

- Return your attention to the first puddle of colour and allow it to transform itself into an object. It may be a simple object such as a cube or a sphere or something more detailed such as a flower or a castle. Again, don't think about it, just allow something to emerge.

- When you can clearly see the object in your first hand, move your attention to your other hand and allow another object to emerge from the second puddle of colour.

- Once the second object is clear, return your attention to the first one and start to investigate it. Is it heavy or light? Weigh it in your hand. Is it hot or cold? If hot, is it burning your hand? If cold, is it uncomfortably so? Is its surface hard or soft, rough or smooth? Imagine yourself running your fingers over it – what does its texture remind you of? If you were to sniff the object, what would it smell like? And if you were to lick it, what would it taste like?

- When you have finished investigating the first object, turn your attention to the second one. Weigh it in your hand. Is it heavier or lighter than the first, or much the same? Is it hot or cold – and how does its temperature compare with that of the first one? Is its surface hard or soft, rough or smooth? What does its texture remind you of? Does it feel more pleasant to the touch than the first object, or less so? If you were to sniff the object, what would it smell like? Is it a more pleasant smell than that of the first object, or is it less pleasant? And if you were to lick it, what would it taste like? Again, is it a more pleasant taste than that of the first object, or is it less so?

Finally, assess which of the two objects feels more comfortable in your hand.

- Once you have got to know your objects in this way, return your attention once more to the first object and ask it what it would like to say to you. Don't think about it . . . just allow its reply to come into your mind. If you want to discuss this with the object, do so. When you have finished your conversation, do the same thing with the second object.

- Then ask the objects whether they have anything they want to say to each other. If a question comes into your mind, based on what the objects have or haven't said, ask it and see if either or both can answer it for you.

- Finally, ask yourself which object do you feel more comfortable with. What have you learned about the two situations? Take your time just to absorb and process the information that you have received.

- When you are completely ready, thank the objects and then allow them to melt back into puddles of colour and allow the puddles to disappear. Turn your hands palm down and very slowly open your eyes and come back into the room.

I remember, some years ago, using this with a client who was having problems in her marriage. She could see no way of resolving them and was thinking of leaving her husband. But she was torn, because she still loved him. It seemed to me that this visualisation might help her to understand her feelings better and come to a decision.

In the hand which represented splitting up, she saw a purplish blue puddle which grew into a flimsy-looking flower with a fresh smell. In the hand which represented staying together, she saw an orange puddle grow into a clover leaf. The clover seemed unbalanced, leaning to one side, and felt uncomfortable in her hand. It had a smoky smell – something she found both reassuring and dangerous. So far, it sounded as though the object representing splitting up would turn out to be the more appealing option.

But when the client invited the clover and the flower to talk to her, something very significant happened. The clover pointed out that the flower was insubstantial, while the flower observed that the clover needed to find a balance. Now, looking at the clover, the client could see that its roots were firm – the only problem was that it was leaning to one side. This gave her the clue she needed as to what had gone wrong in her marriage and enabled her to understand what it was she needed to do to bring it back into balance again. And this, she realised, was what she wanted to do.

In Gestalt psychology there is a technique known as 'chair work' which can help clients to deal with problems they are to do with relationships. The client is asked to sit facing an empty chair and picture the person he or she is having problems with sitting there, and have a conversation with them. After this, the client moves into the empty chair and 'becomes' the other person, expressing that person's views in another conversation. The technique can also be used when someone is in conflict with himself – and, as I have discovered, the 'colour puddle technique' can also be very effective in this respect.

A client whom I was seeing some years ago was having problems with an inner voice which kept telling him that he wasn't working hard enough, that he was lazy and that he would never amount to anything. We did this exercise and he created an object to represent himself in one hand and an object to represent the voice in the other. Having investigated the form of each object and got to know them, he asked them to talk to each other. In my notes I wrote "At the end of the exercise he was unable to put into words what had happened during the exercise but said he knew exactly what it meant". And this understanding helped him, in due course, to dismiss the voice and acknowledge that he was not lazy and always did his best with anything he undertook.

A note for therapists:

If you are using this visualisation with a client, it is helpful to ask him or her to keep up a running commentary so that you know what is happening. Ask whatever questions seem appropriate to you in order to help the client get the most out of the exercise. This is not a rigid exercise – I tend to use it slightly differently every time.

Chapter Ten

Two Versatile Visualisations

I have left these two visualisations until last because, although they are quite different from each other, they are both multi-purpose. Both involve talking (in your mind) to something or somebody that you have formed an image of. The first can be of value when you are troubled by strong, uncomfortable emotions, such as anger, fear or disappointment. The second can help when you feel overwhelmed or confused and need to be able to sort out your thoughts. But they both have uses in other situations so, if you feel that one of them could help you, try it and see.

EXTERNALISING YOUR EMOTIONS

The first visualisation is based on the fact that strong emotions can be felt as physical symptoms – such as tightness in the chest, discomfort in the intestines, or pain in the head or neck.

- Make yourself comfortable and close your eyes.

- Allow yourself to become aware of the emotion that you are feeling. Focus on it and see where in your body you are feeling it. Once you have localised it, allow it to grow very slightly – not too much, don't let it become too uncomfortable.

- Then ask yourself: if the feeling had a colour, what colour would it be?

- When the colour has become clear, ask yourself: if it had a shape, what shape would it be?

- And then: if it had a texture, what would that texture be?

- After that: if it were to make a sound, what would it be?

- And finally: if it had a smell, what would it smell like?

- Take your time over all of these and don't try to think up the answers – just let them arise out of your subconscious mind.

- Now that the feeling is starting to take on a form, ask yourself whether that form feels heavy or light or somewhere in between.

- And then ask yourself whether it is hot or cold, or somewhere in between.

- By this point, you will have developed a pretty good image of your feeling. So now imagine that you are lifting it out of your body and placing it on a surface in front of you – ideally a table, but it can be a chair or even the floor.

- Now you can have a discussion with it. Ask it whatever questions seem appropriate. You may, for example, want to ask why it keeps troubling you or what it wants from you. Don't try to imagine what it will reply, just wait patiently and allow your subconscious mind to provide the answers.

- When you have talked to it and, hopefully, got to know it a little better, ask it what you need to do to turn it into a positive force. If this seems strange, remember that there is a positive aspect to every negative emotion – for example, for anger it could be strength, for fear it could be diligence and for disappointment it could be acceptance or humility. The answer may not come straight away and, while it may be something such as a realisation that there is a particular thing in your life that you need to change, it may not be so straightforward. For example, you may get an answer involving a visualisation such as "you need to bathe me in pink light". In such a case, ask what the pink light signifies, so you understand exactly why you need to do this.

- Once you've got your answer, express your thanks and give the feeling your permission to return to your body on the understanding that it will be less persistent than before and will disappear completely after you have done what it has said you need to do. Then picture the feeling dissolving and, when it has, in your own time, gently open your eyes and come back into the room.

You may need to repeat the exercise a number of times and, if you do, it is likely – assuming that you have been following the guidance it has given you – that what the feeling looks, feels, sounds and smells like will change over time, as will the answers about what you need to do to transform it. Eventually, when it has transformed, you can thank it for its help and stop doing the exercise.

While this visualisation can be used to investigate and resolve a range of unpleasant emotions and feelings, the following visualisation can be used to deal with a variety of situations.

THE CLEARING IN THE WOODS

- Make yourself comfortable, close your eyes and relax. If necessary use the golden light exercise to ensure that you are really relaxed.

- Imagine that you are walking into a wood. It is a beautiful summer's day and the sun is shining through the trees, dappling the path on which you are walking. Become aware of the way the light breeze rustles through the leaves. Alongside the path you may see little woodland flowers, birds and perhaps even rabbits. Continue to walk along the path, enjoying the combination of sunshine and shade.

- After a few minutes you come to a clearing, surrounded by trees. In the middle of the clearing is a large log. It looks old and gives the impression that many people have sat on it over the years.

- Go over to the log and sit down. The log is comfortable to sit on, and you can feel the warm sunshine and the gentle breeze on your skin.

- As you sit on the log, think for a moment or two about the problems you need to resolve. Then just allow yourself to relax.

- Soon you will become aware of someone coming out of the trees behind you and into the clearing. Don't turn around but wait for this person to come over to you and sit beside you on the log.

- As you turn to look at this person you may find that it is someone you know or used to know, someone who looks familiar, or it may be someone that you don't recognise at all. Be aware that, whoever it is, they are there to help you and you can trust them completely. As you start to talk about your problems, you will feel a sense of reassurance, knowing that this person understands what it is that you have been going through.

- Take your time to talk and to listen to what the person has to say. When everything that needs to be said has been said, the other person will get up from the log. After you have thanked them for coming, they will turn and walk back into the woods.

- When the person has gone, you notice that a gift has been left for you on the log. This gift may be absolutely anything – but it will relate in some way to your problems. Pick it up and be aware of how it looks and how it feels in your hand. If you don't immediately see its significance, don't worry – it will come to you. Just be aware that it is yours to keep and that it will help you.

- When you are ready, get up from the log and walk back through the wood, taking your gift with you. As you emerge from the wood, you see in front of you a beautiful, peaceful landscape and you are aware that you are now in a better position to find a resolution to your problems.

- Then, very slowly, in your own time, open your eyes and come back into the room.

This visualisation can also be used to resolve unfinished business. Some years ago I had a client who told me that, when he was a child, a local woman used to look after him while his mother was at work. He was very fond of this woman and, in some ways, was closer to her than to his mother but, after a few years, his family emigrated and he didn't see her again. He often thought of her and, in his thirties, tried to track her down and heard that she had died. The extent of his grief surprised him. I suggested that he do this visualisation, with this woman being the person who came out of the woods to talk to him. He had a long conversation with her and the gift that she left him was, he later told me, something that was very special to him. At the end of the visualisation, he said that he felt that a huge weight had been lifted.

Chapter Eleven

A Note on Manifestation

A lot of people nowadays talk about manifestation – but what exactly does it mean? The Verywell Mind website defines it as making your dreams, goals, and aspirations a reality by believing you can achieve them. And, for a couple of decades or more, various personal development gurus have been advocating using affirmations to bring this about – things such as 'I will do well in my exams' or 'I will find my dream house' or 'I will get the job I want'. The affirmations have to be repeated over and over again, and there is no doubt that, for some people, they work.

One important stipulation when manifesting is that the affirmation and the desire on which it is based have to be specific. Otherwise, as one trainer said "It's like going to a travel agent and saying 'I want to go to hot and sunny'. Yes, you may well end up somewhere hot and sunny but it could be the middle of the Sahara desert, while you were thinking more of the French Riviera."

And this is why visualisation can prove to be better for manifesting your desires than simple affirmations can be. In a visualisation, not only can you put in every detail but you can also manifest the things that will lead up to the final achievement.

For example, if you are manifesting for good exam results, you might think that the best visualisation would be to see yourself celebrating after you have received them. And, certainly, this could help you develop a strong belief that you can pass the exams. But how much more convincing it would be to your subconscious mind if you also visualise yourself working towards your exams and revising – and finding it easy, remembering effortlessly all the information that you need to know. And then you could add a visualisation of the exams themselves, with you looking at the questions and knowing exactly how to answer them, feeling confident in your abilities and feeling none of the stress that is often caused by exams.

So, if there is something you want to manifest, before you do anything else, make a list of the stages involved in that manifestation. In the case of the exams, it would be studying, revising, sitting the exams, and celebrating. In the case of the perfect job, it might be seeing the advertisement, applying for the job, having an interview, receiving the job offer, and actually working in the job.

Once you have your list, for a week or so, spend about five minutes each day visualising the first stage. Then for the next week, spend ten minutes visualising the first two stages. And so on, adding a stage and five minutes each week, until you have a visualisation of the complete process – from studying to celebrating, or from seeing the advertisement to working in the job. And then continue with that visualisation until, hopefully, you achieve your dream.

PART TWO

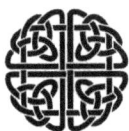

ART

Chapter Twelve

Using Art as a Self-Help Technique

Many of us who had art lessons at school will remember being taught about perspective, composition and colour combinations. What we weren't taught is that art is not just about producing a pretty picture – it is a wonderful way of working with our thoughts and our emotions. How many of us, when angered by something that has happened to us, have scribbled hard on a sheet of paper in order to lessen our frustration? Or perhaps we have drawn caricatures or stick people to represent those who have caused our frustration and then scribbled over them. And, in doing so, we may have realised that it is much easier to express our feelings in this way than by putting them into words.

The psychoanalyst Sigmund Freud, working with

patients in the early twentieth century, observed that many of them were unable to describe in words the dreams that troubled them but were able to express in drawings the emotions that those dreams aroused. And his contemporary, Carl Jung, believed that dreams, art and story-telling could all, through symbolism, provide a link to his patients' unconscious minds. In 1916 he wrote "Often it is necessary to clarify a vague content by giving it a visible form. This can be done by drawing, painting, or modelling. Often the hands know how to solve a riddle with which the intellect has wrestled in vain."

In the 1930s, as the idea of art therapy started to emerge, Mary Huntoon, an artist working at a clinic in Kansas, used art to help patients to process and release emotional problems and trauma. But it was becoming clear that art was something that everyone could benefit from. The psychiatrist Hans Prinzhorn, who died in 1933, certainly believed this, stating that art was a natural way for everyone to achieve good mental health. Bernie Marek, late professor of art therapy at Naropa University in Colorado, wrote "Healing begins when we allow our images the space to be seen and felt."

When used in therapy, art can help patients to analyse and understand their problems. But, as a statement on the website of the American Art Therapy Association makes clear, it can also be used as a therapy in itself because "the creative process involved in making art is healing and life enhancing". And this, of course, makes it very suitable as a self help method. The goal of art therapy, according to therapist Shaun McNiff, is not to find an explanation or a cure: "The goal is to continue to work with [the images] deeply and imaginatively, in order to uncover what our emotions may be trying to teach us." So, if we are prepared to be honest with ourselves and look at what our pictures are telling us and not just what we want to see, we can understand ourselves much better.

When working with his patients, McNiff asks them to speak to their pictures: "Look at the picture carefully. Look deeply . . . as if you are watching another person. Begin to speak by telling this 'other' what you see in it." And when they have done this, they are asked to change roles and respond on behalf of the picture.

In all of this, it is the feelings and the symbolism that are important. In order to benefit from this sort of therapy or self help, you don't have to be 'an artist' – in other words, it doesn't matter at all whether or not you can draw or paint. In fact, sometimes it is better if you can't, because people who are artists will be concerned about getting the perspective and the composition and the colour balance right – about producing a beautiful or an interesting picture – and that is not what this is about at all.

So how can you use art to help yourself? Well, there are two ways. In the first, you can draw or paint images, and in the second you can use images – photographs or artwork – created by other people. We shall look at these in the next two chapters.

Chapter Thirteen

You Don't Have to be an Artist!

In one sense, art is simple because all you need is some paper and some coloured pencils or pens. The best size of paper is probably A4 (21 x 29.7cm) or A5 (14.85 x 21cm) – if it is too big, you may find the prospect of filling it daunting, and if it is too small, you may not be able to express yourself fully.

But, no matter what the size, a blank sheet of paper in itself can be quite daunting so it can help to have a technique you can use to get started. Remember that you are not trying to produce a 'picture' – it doesn't have to represent anything unless you particularly want it to. Indeed, it can just be a scribble if that expresses the way you feel. The picture on the next page was drawn by a client of mine who suffered from claustrophobia.

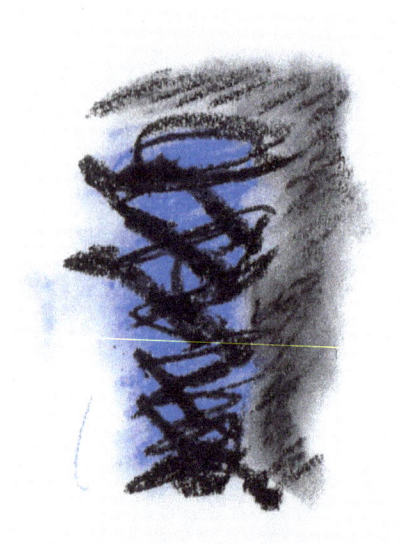

An expression of claustrophobia,
drawn with pastels

Although it's little more than a scribble, it illustrates very clearly what it feels like to be claustrophobic.

STARTING WITH A VISUALISATION

You may find it helpful to use one of the visualisations described in the first section of this book before you start your drawing. For example, you could use the first part of the first visualisation in chapter ten:

- Make yourself comfortable and close your eyes.

- Allow yourself to become aware of the emotion that you are feeling. Focus on it and see where in your body you are feeling it. Once you have localised it, allow it to grow very slightly – not too much, don't let it become too uncomfortable.

- Then ask yourself: if the feeling had a colour, what colour would it be?

- When the colour is clear, ask yourself: if it had a shape, what shape would it be?

- And then: if it had a texture, what would that texture be?

Then, instead of continuing with the exercise, open your eyes and draw the emotion in the way that you have visualised it.

Or you could start by using the 'path round the hill' visualisation described in chapter eight, and then draw what it was that you found on the path – the clue to what is holding you back. It may be that, as you draw, its significance becomes clearer. And, by drawing it in as much detail as you can, you are sending a message to your subconscious mind that you want to understand the meaning of this clue.

Similarly, when you have completed the 'clearing in the wood' visualisation described in chapter ten, you could draw the gift that was left for you by the person with whom you were talking. Again, its significance may become clearer as you draw, and the fact of drawing it may help you to understand more fully what it is trying to tell you.

Whichever 'starter' you use, you may find that you want to add more detail as you go along, or perhaps a background suggests itself to you. As you draw, remain aware of how you are feeling. What thoughts are coming into your mind? You may feel that you want to write some words or phrases on your picture. Just do whatever seems appropriate. Once you have added something to the picture, leave it as it is – don't try to rub anything out or 'correct' it.

STARTING WITH A SHAPE

Another way to get started is to use a simple line or shape and build on it. Have a look at the lines on the next page. Does one of them particularly catch your eye? Or does one of them suggest a particular shape or object to you? Try copying the line and then use that as the start of your drawing.

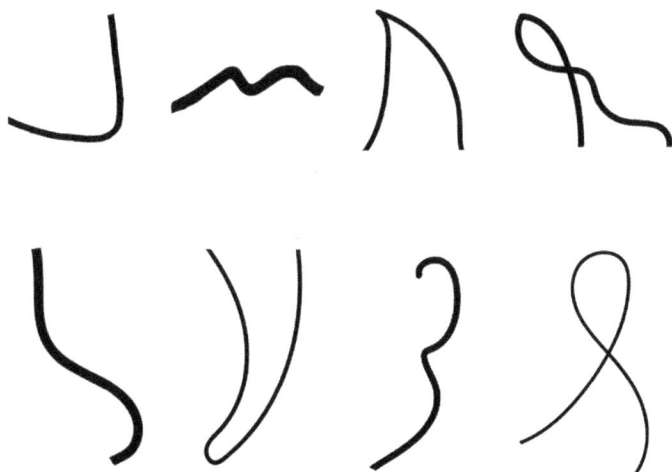

WHAT NEXT?

When you've finished your picture, give it a title and put the date on it. Then put it somewhere safe and, after a few weeks, have a look at it and see whether your feelings about it have changed or whether it seems to be expressing something different. What is the picture telling you?

KEEPING A FEELINGS JOURNAL

If the idea of drawing your feelings appeals to you, you may like to try keeping a feelings journal. For this, you will need a notebook of plain paper, ideally A5 size (14.85 x 21cm).

Then every day, preferably at the same time of day, take ten minutes or so to draw in your journal an expression of how you are feeling, remembering to give it a title and to date it when you have finished. If you can't manage every day, three or four times a week is fine.

After you've been keeping your journal for three or four weeks, look back at what you have drawn. Can you see a pattern of any sort in your emotions or in the way you have expressed them. Does anything jump out at you that didn't before?

Some years ago I had a client who was keeping a feelings journal and, in one of our sessions, we were reviewing it together. We came to a drawing that he had done some months before. It was of a teardrop shape on a black background. At the time, he had said it represented all his sadness and the fact that he was starting to be able to express it. But reviewing it at the later date, when he had been making considerable progress, he saw it quite differently. He described it as a bulb that had been buried in the earth, but had now started to sprout and had the potential to grow into a beautiful plant. He realised now that the point at which he started to be able to express his sadness was also the point when he started to grow out of the darkness. It was, he said, something that gave him confidence in his own abilities to overcome whatever problems he might encounter in the future.

Chapter Fourteen

Looking at Pictures

While drawing pictures is about expressing our feelings in art, looking at pictures can be used to investigate and explore our feelings. To do this, we need to use the picture to tell a story. Let's look at this, using three photographs.

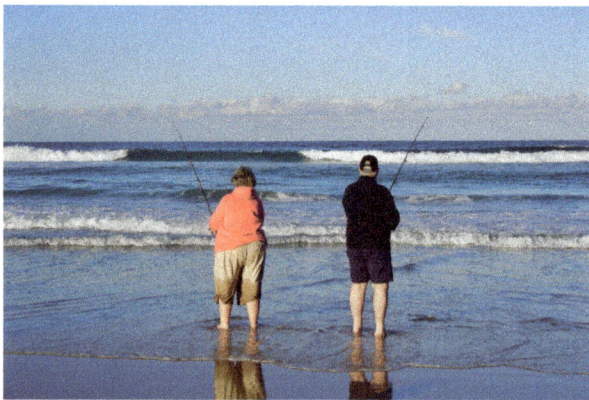

Photo: Fishing by MemoryCatcher on Pixabay

Looking at this image, if you are feeling well emotionally, you might comment on the waves rolling gently onto the beach, the clear sky and the sunshine, the way in which the two people fishing are reflected in the water they're standing in – and the overall feeling would be one of peace and simple pleasures.

But if you were feeling down you might say that here is an old couple who have got nothing better to do than stand in the shallows – where they are unlikely to catch anything – holding on to their fishing rods, for hours on end. And you might note that the ends of the trousers of the person on the left are wet and must be uncomfortable. And so the overall feeling would be one of boredom and discomfort and emptiness.

If you are aware of negative feelings arising when you look at the picture, the next step is to ask yourself how those feelings fit into your life? What is stopping you from feeling peaceful and appreciating simple pleasures? What is boring and uncomfortable in your own life? What can you do to overcome that? And what do you need in order to fill the emptiness? It is important that, in doing this, you are gentle with yourself and allow the answers to come to you, rather than trying to force them.

The next photo, if you look at it when you are feeling well, may tell a story of a lovely walk on a warm summer's day, either on your own or with someone you are fond of. It may include woodland creatures popping out of the undergrowth, and birds singing in the trees. You may be aware of the pleasant smell of the plants around you, and perhaps you imagine running your hand over the bark of some of the trees or pausing to pick up a pebble or a leaf.

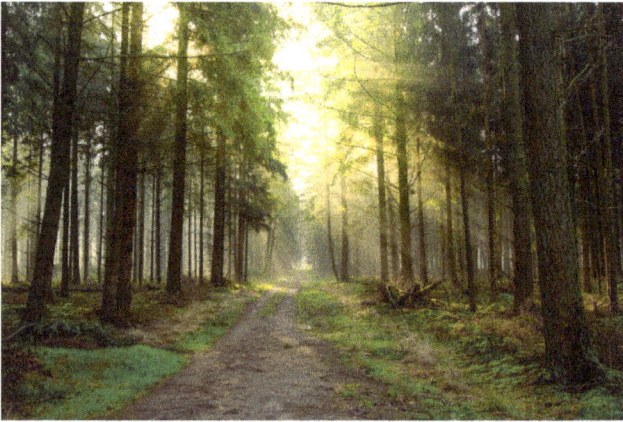

Photo: Forest by Skitterphoto on Pixabay

But if you are feeling down, all you may be aware of is the path disappearing into the distance and how far you are going to have to walk to get to the end. So the overall feeling may be one of exhaustion. And the question would then be: what is it in your life that is causing your exhaustion? And what is it that you are trying to achieve? Is there an easier way of doing it? Are you demanding too much of yourself? And who can you ask for help?

The final photo, like the first, may – if you are feeling well – give you a sense of peace. The water is calm and still, the mist over the lake gives the impression that it is early morning, and the sun shining on the boat suggests that it is going to be a beautiful day. So it may also convey a feeling of hopefulness.

But, if you are feeling low, all you may see is the boat which appears to be abandoned. And your story may be about loneliness or isolation. And, once again, you may need to ask yourself why you are feeling that. Are you lonely? Do you feel abandoned? Is there something you can do about it. Is there someone who can help you?

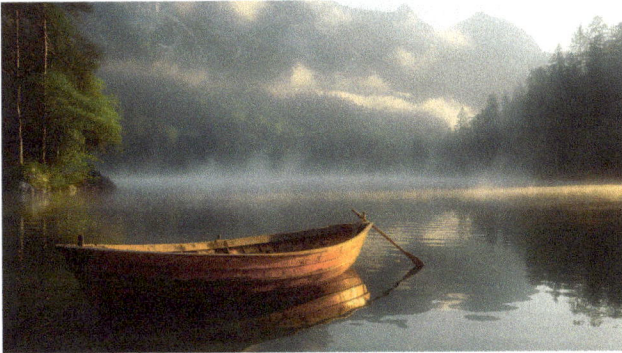

Photo: Tomorrow by Kyraxys on Pixabay

In every case, once you have finished investigating any

negative emotions brought up by the pictures, try to see how else the image might be interpreted – for example, in the pictures we have looked at here, peace, pleasure or hopefulness. And ask yourself how you might convert the one to the other. Because if both the negative and the positive are there in the picture, then the positive can be encouraged to override the negative in your life.

There is, however, another scenario for all or any of these pictures. The image may bring a sense of sadness or yearning. In this case, you may want to ask yourself what it is that you are lacking. Maybe the first image reminds you of happier times and of people who you have lost. The next step would then be to ask yourself whether you have allowed yourself to mourn the loss adequately. What was it that made those earlier times so happy? What do you need to make your life as happy now? And how can you go about finding it?

The second and third images might bring up a yearning for the peace they convey. In this case, the question you need to ask yourself is what is disturbing your peace and what can you do to remedy that. What can you change in your life to make it more peaceful? Do you allow yourself enough personal time or are you too busy rushing around to devote any time to your personal well-being. Half an hour of 'me' time every day can make a lot of difference.

ONE WORD OF WARNING! If you find, at any time, that working with images is bringing up any seriously negative emotions, please stop doing the exercise and consult a professional – either a therapist or a doctor.

FINDING IMAGES TO WORK WITH

So, where can you find images to work with? Well, there are several websites that allow you to download photos for free (for example flickr.com and unsplash.com). But another useful way is to use a deck of tarot cards. A lot of people, when they hear the phrase 'tarot cards' think of the stark drawing of a skeleton with a scythe that, almost inevitably, turns up when someone is reading tarot in a television detective series. But there are many hundreds of different styles of cards, some of which have beautiful artwork. More to the point, unlike the photos we looked at above, tarot cards have been created in order to be interpreted. This means that many of them have a lot more details than a photograph.

One of the decks I use frequently is called the World Spirit Tarot. It was out of print for quite a long time but has recently been reissued and is available from Madame Onça Studios on the Etsy website. My thanks to the deck's creator Lauren Onça O'Leary for permission to reproduce some of the cards here.

The first of these is called The Hierophant.

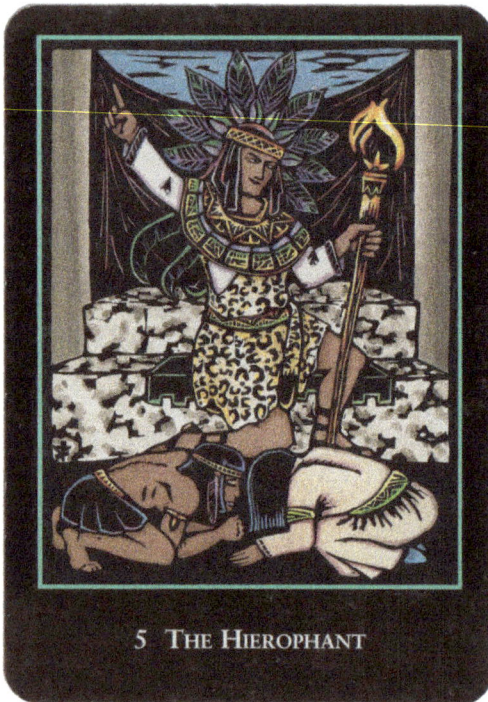

5   THE HIEROPHANT

The word 'hierophant' comes from the Greek, meaning 'one who reveals the holy'. Wikipedia defines the word as "an interpreter of sacred mysteries and arcane principles". So, maybe when we look at this card, we see a teacher expounding great truths to his followers who cower at his feet. Who, then, do we associate with? Are we the hierophant, 'telling it as it is' and brooking no disagreement? Or are we the disciples who blindly follow him and have no words of our own to say or ideas of our own to put forward?

If we are the hierophant, perhaps we need to ask ourselves why we are so sure that we are right about everything. Why do we feel it necessary to be so dogmatic? Does this intimidate other people? And do we feel isolated as a result? Is it just that we are afraid of being wrong or of appearing foolish? And yet, making mistakes is the natural way in which we learn things. If we never make a mistake, we will never learn and never progress. What is this card telling us about ourselves?

If, however, we relate more to the disciples, why are we afraid of speaking up? What is it that we are scared of? How can we overcome that fear?

As always with these pictures, there is another way of looking at this. If we look carefully at the whole card, it may seem that the two disciples, far from being cowed by the hierophant, are having a little chat and a giggle from their crouching position at his feet. They almost look as though they might be playing a game. Whatever it is that they are doing, they are certainly not paying any attention to the hierophant who is doing everything he can to make himself noticed.

With this scenario, are you the hierophant or the disciples? If the former, why do you have to work so hard to be noticed? And why is it so important? If the latter, are you so caught up in your own stuff that you have no time for anyone else? Are you ignoring someone who is trying to relate to you or to tell you something important?

Of course, you might have another interpretation altogether – when you are working with pictures, it is your interpretation that counts, not anyone else's. And you may well look at a picture on one day and interpret it in one way and, a few weeks later, interpret it in a completely different way, depending on what is going on in your life at that moment.

The next card is the three of swords (the suits in tarot decks are different from the suits in ordinary playing cards).

What is the story here? A figure (possibly a woman) cowers in the foreground. Three daggers pin a scroll to the wall. Round the corner we see the reflection of another figure, looking the other way. Who do we relate to – the terrified woman or the person looking the other way? And, if we are the terrified woman, what are we so afraid of? The only weapons to be seen are stuck in the wall. No one has been stabbed or injured in any way. And, if necessary, she could pull one of the daggers out of the wall and use it to defend herself. Are we, like her, cowering in fear rather than looking around to see how we can stand up for ourselves?

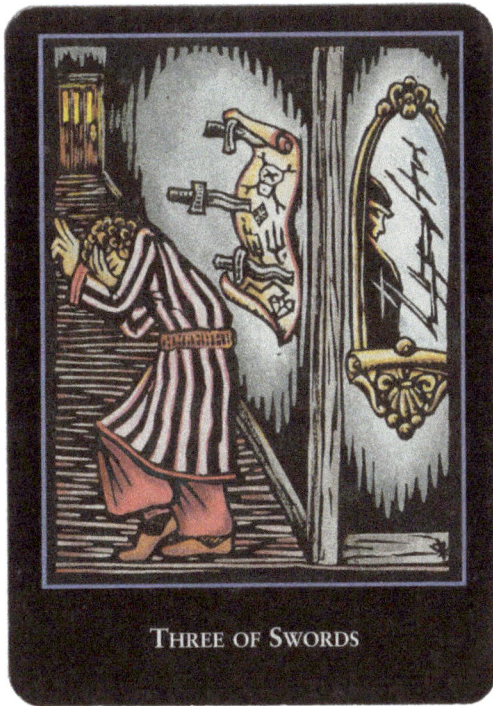

THREE OF SWORDS

And what about the scroll itself? It is hard to see what is on it, but it could be something that would help the woman. Perhaps it is a map that will show her how to reach a place of safety. Why doesn't she look at it to see

what it might offer? It might even show her that, at the
end of the corridor, there is a door (which we can see if we
look closely at the card). But the woman seems unaware
of it. What is stopping her from making her escape? Is it
lack of confidence in her ability to do so? And – since the
person reflected in the mirror looks fairly benign, why isn't
she asking for help? Is it because she feels unable to trust
anyone?

But what if we relate not to the fearful woman but to the
person in the mirror? Why are we just standing there out
of sight and not offering help? Is it simply that we trust
the woman to find her own way out of the situation? Is
it that we don't want to get involved? Is it that we don't
really care? What are our motives for doing nothing when
we could help?

Again, you may well see a different interpretation,
depending on what is happening in your life at the
moment.

The third card is from the same suit.

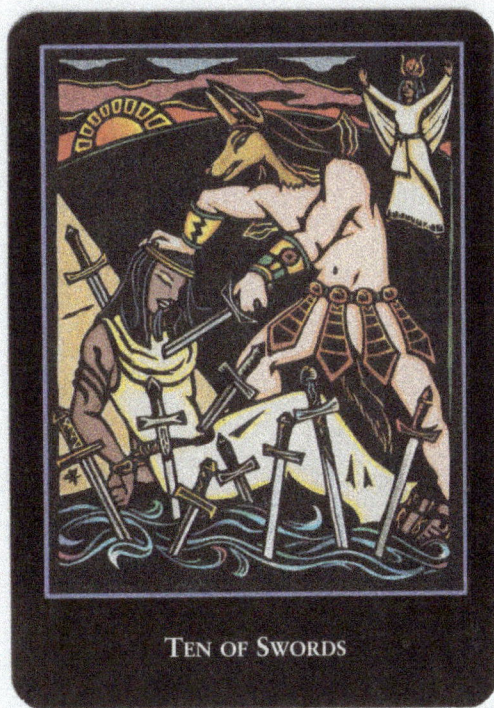

TEN OF SWORDS

It shows a woman who has been run through by swords, one of which is being held by a figure who looks like the Egyptian jackal-headed god, Anubis, What are we to make of this?

Perhaps your immediate perception is that Anubis has stabbed her, determined to put an end to her with not just one but several swords. She looks as though she has given up and is ready to die. In the background we can see the sun and an angel, suggesting that her sun is setting and the angel is waiting to take her into heaven.

Or perhaps there is another way of looking at it. If you are feeling good, if your life is going well, maybe you see the angel as coming to help the woman, to rescue her from Anubis. But what if she doesn't need rescuing? What if Anubis, rather than stabbing her, is removing the swords from her body in an effort to heal her? And what if the sun, rather than setting, is rising on a new day, which the angel is there to proclaim?

Once again, we need to examine our reactions to the image. If we saw the woman as dying from a vicious attack, giving up because she had no fight left, we have to ask ourselves what it is that we feel we have to give up on. And if it is something that we don't want to give up, is there someone who can help us get through this dark patch – is there an Anubis who can help us to recover from whatever it is that has attacked us or certain aspects of our lives? Is there someone or something who can, metaphorically, remove the swords and allow us to experience the new day?

The role of images in all of this is to make us aware of our feelings – feelings that we might be suppressing or misinterpreting or not understanding fully. But, after that, it is important to start to question ourselves as to what we need to do – what is the positive interpretation of the picture, and how do we get there from where we are?

Chapter Fifteen

The Wonder of Colour

Many people have a favourite colour. The chances are that you have, too. But have you ever stopped to wonder why it is your favourite? Is it a colour that looks good on you, so you like to wear it? Or perhaps it reminds you of somebody or something. Or is there just something about it that makes you feel good?

Many studies have been done over the years into people's reactions to different colours. In one, it was found that people with a doctor's appointment who were asked to wait in a blue room were far more patient and relaxed about the wait than others who were shown into a yellow room.

Other studies have shown that people tend to associate the colour green with tranquillity, contentment, cleanliness, hope and renewal. But it is a very personal thing. At one time there was a popular superstition that green was unlucky. And I remember being in a card shop some years ago and hearing a lady saying that she had found a card she liked but wouldn't buy it because it came with a green envelope and "I hate green".

Similarly, studies have shown that people associate yellow with feelings of happiness and optimism but, as the waiting room experiment shows, an excess of yellow (in this case, all the walls painted in that colour) can increase people's levels of anxiety. However, once again, it is a personal thing. I love the colour yellow – it is one of my two favourites. But my mother disliked it so, in our house when I was growing up, we didn't wear yellow and there were no yellow walls or furnishings. I once asked my mother why she was so averse to yellow, and she didn't know. She just knew that she didn't like it.

In the late nineteenth century, neurologists began speculating that different colours affected our nervous systems in different ways. And, for a number of years, scientists (and a few quacks) promoted a variety of forms of colour therapy in which light was shone through glass of different colours onto the patients' bodies. No benefit was ever proved – possibly because no account was taken of patients' individual preferences.

However, recent studies have gone some way to vindicate these early promoters of colour therapy. Kathy Willis, professor of biodiversity at Oxford University, in her book *Good Nature* (Bloomsbury, 2024) looks at research into the effect that interacting with nature has on our minds and bodies. And it seems that colour is a major factor in this, with plants that have leaves that are green and white or flowers that are white or yellow having the greatest effect, lowering heart rate, blood pressure and the level of stress hormones, and resulting in greater calmness and clearer thinking.

And, strange as it may seem, colours may affect us even if we, as humans, can't see them (although some insects can). Light travels in waves, red having the longest wavelength and violet the shortest. We are frequently warned about ultraviolet light which has a wavelength shorter than violet and which we can't see but which, nonetheless, can affect our skin and cause sunburn. And, at the other end of the specturm, infrared light, which has a wavelength longer than red, is also invisible but can be perceived as heat.

A colour therapist told me of an experiment that was done some years ago with a group of blind people, some of whom had been blind from birth. A selection of silk scarves – all identical apart from their colours – were passed from person to person. Every now and again the

experimenter would say "If you think you're holding a
red scarf, please hold it up". Or "If you think you're
holding a green scarf . . ." through all the colours that
were circulating. And in the majority of cases, the correct
colours were held up. At one point the experimenter asked
what it was that made those who had correctly identified
the yellow scarves so sure of their identification. The
answer was immediate – yellow felt somehow 'stickier'
than the other colours.

So working with colour is not just about the way it looks
to your eye. It's also about the feelings and sensations it
arouses. And remember, too, that every colour has many
shades (as the paint companies delight in reminding us in
their advertisements). Navy blue is likely to evoke quite
different feelings from soft baby blue, and bottle green is
unlikely to conjure up the same feelings or images as grass
green or moss green. In the visualisations that follow, try
not to use your logical mind to tell you what the colours
mean (for example, red for anger or yellow for happiness)
but just allow yourself to be aware of what they mean to
you at that precise moment. What feelings do they evoke?
Do they make you feel happy . . . sad . . . excited . . . anxious
. . . confident . . . nervous? Take your time and allow the
feelings to emerge.

FINDING OUR OWN COLOURS

The basis of this exercise is a very simple visualisation. Once you have done it a few times, you may not even need to shut your eyes to do it. Just imagine that you are surrounded by a cocoon of light. Then look to see what colour the light is. It is unlikely to be one colour. You will see swirls of different shades in the cocoon. Note where the various colours are and allow yourself to understand what those colours mean to you at that point. Don't think about it. Just let the meaning come to you. And it won't be the same every time - on one occasion you may be aware of a red colour that represents love and the concern you have for someone close to you. But on another occasion the same shade of red may be associated with anger or with an excess of energy or enthusiasm.

The exercise can be a fairly accurate representation of your feelings at any one time and it may bring up those feelings before you're actually aware of them. On one occasion some years ago, I had become stuck with a particular piece of work I was doing and my light had been various shades of brown and grey for some weeks. Then, one morning, I had a look at it and it was peach coloured with some light blue and pink and I realised that it was the colour of sunrise and it was indicating to me that I was now ready to tackle the piece of work again – which I did, successfully.

WHAT'S MISSING?

Not only can the visualisation of our own colours indicate to us what is going on in our emotional world, but it can also tell us what we need. When you have finished looking at your colours and interpreting them, ask yourself "What – if anything – is missing?" The answer may be that there is nothing missing. Or you may become aware that there is a colour that you need. For example, if you are feeling tired, you may need some red. Or if you are anxious, you may need a soft blue. But, once again, it is important to remember that the colour you need is not necessarily the obvious one – red for energy, blue for relaxation – but the colour that your body and your subconscious mind tell you that you need. You may discover, for example, that you need a shade of violet or a very pale peach or a pearly grey. Just trust your senses.

Once you have decided what it is that is lacking, you can use another visualisation to provide it.

BRINGING IN A NEEDED COLOUR

- As usual, sit comfortably, close your eyes and relax.

- And imagine that you're in a small wooded valley, walking beside a little river. The water is sparkling and very clear – you can see the pebbles on the river bed and little fish as they dart round in the water.

- Up ahead of you, you can see a waterfall. Walk towards it. And, as you do so, you will become aware that there is a small recess behind it, right next to the path you are on.

- Step in there and turn around so that you are looking back at the river and the valley through the waterfall.

- As you stand there, be aware that the water is changing into pure energy and the colour of the waterfall is changing to the colour that you need. Step into it and let it pour over you. Be aware of how it feels. Stay there for as long as you want to.

- When you have taken as much colour as you need,

thank the waterfall and step out of it. Then watch it change back into sparkling water before you return to the path and walk back along the valley. Be aware of any differences you feel as you walk.

- Then slowly allow the scene to fade from your mind before opening your eyes and coming back into the room.

PART THREE

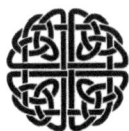

DREAMS

.

Chapter Sixteen

Understanding Your Dreams

We all dream. And most of us remember some of our dreams. Even if you tend not to remember your dreams very well, you can train yourself to do so by writing down as much as you *can* remember as soon as you wake up. Because dreams are important. In the previous chapters we have looked at using images that we either consciously create or decide to use. But the imagery of dreams comes directly from the subconscious mind and can draw our attention to things that we need to deal with.

Those of us who were told Bible stories as children will probably remember the tale of the Egyptian Pharaoh who dreamed about seven fat cows and then seven skinny cows and was told by Joseph that this meant that there would be seven years with good harvests followed by seven years of famine. In the Bible and other sacred scriptures and stories, the dreams always have to be interpreted by a wise man or wise woman. But, actually, it is we ourselves who can best interpret and use our dreams. However, like pictures, they can be interpreted in many different ways – and they don't always mean what we think they do. This is why it is best to avoid ready-made interpretations that you can find in books and on websites. For example, if you search online for the interpretation of a dream in which you are working in a laboratory, you will discover a wealth of meanings – that you are experimenting with your creative abilities or with your beliefs or with a relationship, or that you are going through a transformation, or that you need to resolve a problem that was of your own making, or that there has been a misunderstanding . . . the list goes on and on. And, while your dream might have one of these meanings, it may mean something else entirely – or, of course, your brain may just be recalling (in a garbled way) an episode of *Bones* that you saw last night on the television.

Most of us, I suspect, have had a dream in which we are late for a meeting or an exam or some other important appointment and we just can't find our way to the place where we are meant to be. It is a classic anxiety dream and, very often, it is quite easy to work out what it is that we are nervous about. But sometimes it is not so obvious. It can prove worthwhile, however, if you have this dream, to take a little time to look at what is going on in your life and ask yourself what it is that you are scared you might not be able to achieve.

If you have had a dream that was disturbing or seems as though it may have a deeper meaning, there is an exercise that may offer enlightenment.

Sit comfortably and shut your eyes. Try to remember how the dream started. Then allow it to progress, as it did when you were asleep – except, this time, you know that it is a dream. As the dream progresses, give a running commentary out loud (it is helpful if you can record this). Make sure you describe not just what is happening but how you are feeling.

For example, someone may describe her dream as: "I'm walking down this dark corridor with doors on either side. And I'm feeling scared because I don't know what's on the other side of those doors. The corridor is very long – I can't see the end of it – but it's an effort to walk and I'm only moving very slowly."

When you get to the end of the dream, allow it to fade and then open your eyes and make a note of what you think the dream may be about.

Now shut your eyes again and pick another viewpoint

to see the dream from. If there was another person or an animal in the dream, you may want to choose them. Or you may feel drawn to an inanimate object. In the example above, the dreamer might choose the corridor itself, or somebody or something behind one of the doors in the corridor. Then go through the exercise again, giving a running commentary from the other viewpoint.

For example, as the corridor it might be something along the lines of "This woman is disturbing me – it's night time and I've had people walking up and down all day and I want to rest. But she is insisting on walking along very slowly and she is not getting anywhere. Why can't she go into one of my rooms or get a move on? I feel as though she doesn't trust me."

Once again, when you get to the end of the dream, allow it to fade and then open your eyes.

Now listen to your running commentaries and ask yourself whether the first one – the one from your viewpoint – tallies with the second one. In the example given, the dreamer is scared of the corridor but, after hearing the second running commentary, it seems that there is no need for this. So what can be deduced from this? Perhaps the dreamer has been trying to do something in her life that she is scared of doing and, because of her hesitation, has been finding it really hard. Perhaps the answer is for her to look at whether there is any valid reason for being scared, whether she really wants to do whatever it is, and – if she does want to – how she might better equip herself to do it. What is the corridor trying to tell her? Perhaps she needs to step back and take a break from the task. If she did, would the corridor seem less scary to her when she returned?

I remember one woman who told me about a disturbing dream she had had. In it, she had come home after an evening out to find her kitchen had been trashed. Now this was a woman whose home was immaculate and for her to find her beautiful kitchen in this state was very distressing. All the contents of the fridge had been taken out and thrown on the floor and the door of the fridge was hanging open. As she described the dream from her point of view, I could hear in her voice how much it had affected her. But, when she started to describe it from the viewpoint of the fridge, her tone was quite different. The fridge explained gently and clearly that sometimes we would like to keep things behind closed doors but eventually we have to confront them. The eggs that had been thrown onto the floor had smashed but "you can't make an omelette without breaking eggs". Eventually it became clear what the dream was about. She had been in a relationship for several months but now her partner had been offered a new job, entailing a move to another part of the country, and she had to decide whether to go with him or whether to stay in the home she loved. She had been putting off making the decision because, whichever choice she made, there would be loss. But the dream made it clear that it was time for her to confess her ambivalence to her partner and come to a decision.

Finally, a note about lucid dreaming. This is when, in a dream, you become aware that you are dreaming. This is very valuable because it allows you to control the dream and, if it is scary, to bring it to a comfortable ending. The Jungian psychotherapist Charlie Morley offers a free online course on lucid dreaming here:

https://www.awakeacademy.org/course/free-lucid-dreaming/

But it is not just the ability to control the dream that makes lucid dreaming valuable. It can also enable you to interact with the images that your subconscious mind is presenting to you. For example, in the dream quoted above, where the woman found her kitchen trashed, she could, in a lucid dream, have asked the fridge what had happened and why. Similarly, in the dream where the woman was walking down the corridor, she could have asked the various doors "What is behind you? What will happen if I open you?", or she could have asked the corridor "What do I need to do to get out of here?".

Our subconscious minds are constantly sending us messages. It is up to us to find a way in which we can interpret them to help us live our lives in a more satisfactory way.

FINDING A THERAPIST

The following sites list qualified therapists, many of whom offer creative therapies (such as art and visualisation). However, if you specifically want to see an art therapist, go to the site of the BAAT in the UK or the AATA in the USA.

UK

British Association for Counselling and Psychotherapy:
https://www.bacp.co.uk/

UK Council for Psychotherapy:
https://www.psychotherapy.org.uk/

National Counselling and Psychotherapy Society:
https://ncps.com/counselling-directory

Psychology Today:
https://www.psychologytoday.com/gb/counselling

Counselling Directory:

https://www.counselling-directory.org.uk/

Mind:

https://www.mind.org.uk/information-support/local-minds/
(low cost counselling, but some Mind counsellors may still be in training)

British Association of Art Therapists:

https://baat.org/find-an-art-therapist/

USA

Psychology Today:

https://www.psychologytoday.com/us/therapists

Therapist: https://therapist.com/

American Art Therapy Association:

https://arttherapy.org/art-therapist-locator/

OTHER COUNTRIES

Psychology Today:

https://www.psychologytoday.com/intl
(click on 'INTL' next to the globe icon top right and then choose the country)

OTHER BOOKS BY RUTH LEVER KIDSON

Acupuncture:

What it is, how it works and how it can help you

Hypnotherapy:

Everything you need to know about hypnosis and how it

can help you